Toddler

Toilet

#1 Consumer Guide for Choosing The Best

Potty Seats for Toddler

Phil Jane

ISBN: 978-1-63750-252-5

Table of Contents

Introduction

Potty training is among the things that provide a new mother or father with an enormous concern. Who must be in-charge, when is the correct time to begin it, how do all of us teach children to make use of the toilet independently, with little or no supervision?

This book is about the utilization of Toilet training seats, the basic facts to consider when buying toilet seats, and a brief review on what I consider the best toilet training seat in the marketplace.

There are several guide online about potty training for kids, no matter the technique, the use of potty training seat or toilet training seat is usually imperative, and the end objective remains the same; ensuring kids use the toilet at the correct time with little or no guidance.

Potty training seat was created specifically for old kids;

antique 3 and above, whilst toilet chair is created for small children beneath age 3, though it is quite feasible to employ a house training chair for children more youthful than 3, It isn't really recommended to take this action, especially intended for the child's security.

It has been proven that kids who also fall from toilet chair usually end up with some kind of anxiety for it's utilization in the future. If you have a more youthful child (above age three, then you definitely should find out about potty seat).

Majority of parents might opt for toilet training chair over toilet seat since it's simpler to just get rid of the poo when a child has pooed, than needing to clean the potty seat once in a while. Apart from protection and the strain for cleaning the toilet seat, both items are just about a similar thing.

There comes a period when you are potty training, the

potty seat is more relevant because as a child, it offers the exact comfort as a toilet seat in a standard toilet. A potty seat is necessary especially when it fits upon the best toilet.

Potty seats are extremely beneficial to have readily available for touring as well as when out in public areas or in other's homes too. Nevertheless, there are so many to select from and it could be difficult to determine which may be the better to purchase for your kid.

You need to ensure they are comfortable and your kid feels protected on it, and also ensure it is functional and simple to use as well. Plus, often children become very mounted on their toilet chair because it is exactly what they grew up to know plus they might not want to use another thing.

However, obtaining a toilet seat that has an equal pattern

or similar design can get things easier. Probably choosing a toilet chair that is definitely cushioned, depending on what your son or daughter desires, and one that can go directly to the toilet successfully each and every time is important. We will understand why and also have produced this whole section upon toilet chair tips and resources to assist choose the best toilet seat pertaining to your kid.

Chapter 1

Toddler Potty Seat

Potty seats are an essential tool to have in the toilet when schooling children. Every toilet of the home is to be maintained so the kid may use any kind of toilet when they have to, plus they have to be available as well.

Toilet seats are to be located right simply by the toilet; therefore, the child can simply grab it. In any event, the potty seat is vital to ensure a kid may use the toilet easily and seems comfy while carrying it out too.

There is a big selection of toilet seats open to fit every single child's needs, as well as their particular likes as well.

Potty seats can be purchased in:

- foldable toilet seats

- travel toilet seats

- smooth toilet seats

- flip toilet seats

The selection above means that there is surely something for everybody as required. Remember again that there must be a potty chair at home, therefore using a couple of different types work as well, or having different styles on may work to motivate your son or daughter to use, given that they can easily see common character types or designs in each space of the home.

Foldable toilet seats and travel potty seats are virtually identical. The foldable toilet seats can be folded up nicely and used for travel as well. They will include fun heroes that children like, such as Dora, Diego, Blues Hints,

Moana and even Elmo. They are extremely light-weight and fit perfectly on the best toilet, therefore a kid can sit easily. The travel potty seats come in a number of designs too, some are inflatable for super easy storage space and travel, while some also collapse up and are padded too.

Smooth toilet seats are padded and again match neatly in the starting of the toilet. You will find this as a private and excellent potty meant for smaller kids that require to carry on when heading out or children that require that extra security with all the toilet. These types have a great time character type attached to them, along with shiny colors and styles too.

The flip family toilet seats replace the existing toilet chair in the toilet, so that there surely is a smaller sized toilet designed for children. You have the cover and a chair with a smaller sized starting that may be flipped when adults require the toilet. They are ideal for kids that might already become toilet qualified but remain too little to match upon a normal toilet. They are done in a number of sizes to match different size lavatories too.

House training doesn't have to become nerve-racking; it's all within your strategy. In the event that you make it all fun just for your son or daughter, he or she could be more reactive and be taught in a shorter time frame.

Chapter 2

Potty Seat vs Potty Chair

When searching for toilet training items you want as much information as you possibly can, to make an informed decision. All of us thus need to understand there are recommendations about how to help make the choice among a toilet chair or toilet seat.

The difference between a Toilet Seat and Toilet Chair initially appear to be a simple question to answer, in most cases the variations are a little more included. Our main focus usually is to offer you enough quality information to help make the best decision for your loved ones, and you must consider a number of different factors to choose, which is the ideal fit to get your loved ones. Additionally, you may have questions like, "Why must I use one on the other"? One of the ways to answer the question is to;

✓ *Know what your son or daughter requirements are.*

✓ *Know what your son or daughter loves.*

This really is dependent upon a number of different aspects, such as, what exactly will work perfectly for your loved ones and what your requirements, needs, and wants are.

What may be ideal for just one family members doesn't invariably imply that it is befitting for yours; honestly, it's dependent upon your family's requirements and desires.

Following this book, you might arrive at the final outcome that both can be useful tools to work with you in house training your tot. The easiest description of both would be that the toilet chair is certainly a stand-alone product that is totally not different from a toilet, and a toilet seat is usually a fixed addition to your existing toilet seat, or can change it completely and can develop change with your son or daughter.

There are benefits and drawbacks concerning all sorts of item that is usually on the marketplace. We cover most of them to enable you make the very best decision pertaining to your loved ones.

Firstly, we can cover professionally a lot of the aspects regarding the toilet seat. Toilet Seats are portable and most of them are light-weight enough, meant for your son or daughter to have the ability to move it themselves. Toilet Seats can be found with tempting fun sizes and shapes, some having a musical feature.

Fun people can embellish the toilet seat and this can be considered an extremely motivating element to your child. The fantastic designs could be aesthetically encouraging to your child and this can be an important aspect to consider as kids of young age group have a tendency to relate more effectively with what is visually activated.

So, in the event that your son or daughter is usually enthralled with pets or a favorite personality, viewing this for the seat may be the extra drive that your son or daughter needs to deal with this next thing in their advancement.

A few of these seats are multi-purpose with tub themed seats that are ideal for your little knight in shining armor or your little princess. coordinating in nearly every decorating scheme. These toilet seats can be changed into a rocking seat designed for your son or daughter to use as they grow in all important stage of advancement. A few of these toilet chairs feature toilet paper and holder that may be removed too.

Potty Seats are kid size, that allows their small feet to have the ability to reach the ground, which usually motivate a far more organic toilet position that will aid all of them in generating a highly effective removal of their particular waste materials.

Toilet Seat encourages independency: At this time of advancement, children have a tendency to test their particular limitations and they are craving to become relatively independent, which when utilizing a toilet chair, they don't really have to require assistance.

Potty Seats:

- There is definitely no transition period with choosing toilet seats.
- It helps you to save the additional expenditure on buying two products i.e. potty chair and potty seat.

- With a toilet seat, there is absolutely no tidy up process to cope with, everything you need to do is usually flushed in the toilet.

Toilet is too much for kids to have the ability to access alone, they'll need assistance via the caregiver or one step stool; so, a child must grow to have the ability to grip something firmly, enabling their sphincter muscles to unwind and giving the ability to effectively utilize the restroom. But it should be noted that the potty seats need to be eliminated for a grown-up to utilize it, which may be of concern if a visitor or various other family are utilizing the toilet.

There are many different facets to either selecting a toilet chair or toilet seat and this truly is dependent upon what's the very best fit just for your loved ones' environment. Though through experience, we have found that utilizing a toilet chair first then shifting into the toilet seat supplies the child with the building blocks of using the toilet.

Therefore, the very best plan of action is usually to hire both wonderful equipment to make sure that your child can be encouraged and has choices to choose from, as long as you, the mother or father, are comfortable with it. I hope you have been offered enough useful information that you should have the ability to make an informed decision.

Potty Chairs

- Most are portable and may be relocated throughout your house, but some could be big and bulky (if space can be an issue, a potty chair is probably not befitting your loved ones).

  For kids:

- They may practice heading the toilet as they grow,

i.e. they have the ability to independently go to the toilet when the need arises. But at the start, you must eliminate out the waste and clean the potty chair after every use.

- There is likely to be a transitional period for the toddler to get accustomed to using the "Big Girl or Boy Toilet".

C h a p t e r   3

Typs of Potty

Even though lots of economic products could make life simpler, the must have item for toilet training is definitely a toilet. In the past, a simple container or dish sufficed for everybody, however, the added comfort and interesting shades of commercial brands enhance small children inspiration.

Two Fundamental Types of Economic Potties:

1. Potty Seats: They may be self-contained models that take a seat on the ground. These are low enough to improve children's emotions of protection and boost a toddler's interest.The drawback is usually a detachable dish which should be transported towards the toilet,

purged and rinsed after every use of it. Also, some children have a problem with the change-over from the potty seat to the standard toilet.

2. Toilet Seats: They may be mounted on the chair of a normal toilet, developing a smaller sized starting, therefore, children avoid fall in. Several small children like the sensation to be developed that originates from using the toilet like old siblings and parents, however, many youngsters fear so much the elevation. Climbing up can be hard, and a frightening fall can confuse training.

Features to Consider before Buying

1. Stability -- The bottom of the toilet chair should be in the least width at the very top for small children and wider at the bottom for the purpose of babies.

2. Splash Guards -- Although dash guards are a benefit intended for sanitation simply by directing a blast of

urine, which usually is particularly helpful for males. Many tots finish up with an agonizing bump sooner or later, and will not want to visit near the toilet afterward. Rising more than a dash safeguard to log off the toilet chair can be difficult enough to result in a fall so splash protects should be cushioned or removable. Normally, ensure there can be an inch between your splash safeguard and the infant's crotch.

3. Security - Toilet seats ought to fasten towards the toilet securely. Examine the grips.

4. Potty Dish -- Bigger is way better for avoiding spills. The dish ought to be easy to eliminate to ensure that small children may vacant all of them independently.

5. Chair -- A chilly, hard toilet chair is definitely less welcoming when compared to a smooth one. Choose a model having a padded chair.

6. Armrests -- If toilet chair has arm sits, children can

automatically grab one and lean onto it as they sit back, which can trigger the seat to overturn. Prevent them.

7. Stepping stool -- Some potty chairs convert to toilet seats, which could cut costs later on, such as the Multi-Function Potties.

8. Portability - A few toilet chair and seats collapse straight down for journeying. Make sure that the hinges are stuffy therefore the device refuses to collapse during normal use. Several children totally reject a single toilet, declining even to look close to this, yet are extremely taken with another brand.

Chapter 4

Types of Todller Potty seats

Toilet training seats can be purchased in a multitude of styles to match almost every child preference or household necessity. Let's check out a few of the most typical types of toilet schooling seats.

Versatile

Buying house training chair that does everything? A versatile model is usually a great choice. These innovative toilet teaching seats have got a fold-out design with an integral stage feces, and several have holders for children to hold to while earning their method to the very best. However, it is critical to remember that this design offers a more substantial impact than others. If you have limited space, storage space is actually a concern.

Traditional

They are generally manufactured from plastic material, with curved seats to improve comfort and promote right positioning. Many traditional toilet training seats feature plastic undersides or flexible "hands" to avoid sliding, and the small size makes it easy to shop.

Hinged

When you have a high-traffic toilet and may do without the trouble of getting to eliminate a toilet schooling chair too many times each day, a hinged model might be your very best bet. These types of innovative seats feature an adult-size chair underneath and another toilet training chair at the top, both of which run with the same hinge. Many also include a cover having a depressive disorder which means that your kiddo's chair rests safely in the cover you definitely use. The largest disadvantage of this kind of toilet chair can be that you will need to displace your whole toilet chair, but also for good sized family members, the capability of this design could be worthwhile.

Flexible fit

A small number of toilet teaching seats provide an adaptable fit to support different toilet sizes. As the actual form and size of the chair stay the same, hands or prongs on the lower end of the chair can be modified to provide a snug in shape that doesn't change or move. Some possess a call you can use to get the hands in or out, while some have prongs that are altered by hand. In any event, versions that provide a changeable match are remarkably convenient, particularly if you need to consider the chair along for sleepovers with the grandma and grandpa or outings to a friend's house.

Cushioned

In the event that comfort is vital, a cushioned potty-training chair can be a choice worth taking into consideration. Whilst standard versions routinely have a built-in coating of cushioning protected with plastic material, others present detachable soft touch pads. If you are considering investing in a cushioned housebreaking chair, be aware that this design can be considerably harder to keep clean than solid models.

Match

Toilet containers come in a variety of sizes and shapes. The most frequent are elongated, with circular coming in a detailed second. Generally, elongated containers measure around 18.625 inches and more, whilst round toilet bowls measure 16.75 inches or less. Selecting a toilet training chair that carefully fits your toilet's sizes is essential to attaining a good suit, so do not forget to factor this into the decision-making process.

Travel

Although the common potty training chair is simple enough to take with you, models that are designed for travelling are undeniably hassle-free. These generally come in another of two designs: fold-up or convertible.

Fold-up travel toilet training seats fold little enough to match into a diaper bag and therefore are perfect for journeying light.

Transformable models look like a normal toilet training chair with fold-out legs and may be utilized and an appropriate plastic material bag like a stand-alone toilet chair is ideal for street trips or stowing in the automobile.

Chapter 5

Considering Buying a Toilet Seat?

With a lot of potties to select from, how will you understand which to buy?

Preferably, the results of most potties ought to be the same, however, there are specific distinguishable features that produce a few seats much better than the rest, greatly differing from the normal.

This is a set of points that you should think about to make sure you get the best of your expense.

Standalone or chair reducer

You can find two types of toilet instructors; standalone rest by itself on to the floor and is obtainable by your son or daughter while chair reducers offer usage of regular toilet seats by lowering how big the adult seats are.

Is this durable and correctly suits your son or daughter or on the toilet?

Protection is the primary concern; your son or daughter need to feel secure and so they don't spook themselves back to diapers.

Is it user-friendly for your son or daughter?

Dealing privately to balance upon can truly add towards the sense of basic safety whilst concurrently also which makes it simpler for the young child to get on and off.

Does it include cushion seats?

These types provide additional comfort and also to allure your son or daughter to maintain returning and continue use.

✓ Is movability a key point for you? - Hassle-free moving of potty chair whether from room to room or for travel purposes need be durable however it should have lightweight seats.

✓ Will it feature splash protects? - These types of preventing unneeded clutter, children splashing on to the floor or their clothing is only going to improve your trouble for cleaning.

✓ What unique features will it include? Sound files, tunes, compartments pertaining to books or playthings are additional features to help encourage your son or daughter to invest in making use of potty.

✓ Does this include extra accessories? Seats come with step bar stools which makes it simpler for the young children to reach the toilet or the kitchen sink for self sufficiency.

Does it add a high back again?

Chances are that your son or daughter would spend an extended time period while pooping thus she or he must become comfortably sitting - in addition, they demand simpler bowel motions.

Chapter 6

How to Know a Perfect Potty Seat

Probably one of the most elementary elements in selecting your potty seat is as easy as asking if the potty your son or daughter usually uses is focused mainly on that child, or if additional family members and guests will use it?

Flip Family Members potty Seats:

If the kid solely uses the toilet, a semi-permanent toilet seat may be your best option for you personally. You have got many choices of semi-permanent toilet seats available, many of these are available on several online stores.

These types of potty seats are to displace the existing toilet seat, it is all comfortable while a grown-up toilet seat is not for infants. It has become popular within the last couple of years. A few Turn Toilet Potty Chair use a hidden-in-the-lid, child-sized toilet seat and a great incentive system; these types can certainly end up being elevated and reduced simply by your son or daughter. You may appreciate the concealed nature of the kid chair - and that there surely is simply no safeguard to stab you in the trunk!

These toilet seats can be purchased in traditional and elongated sizes and can be employed by possibly a grown-up or a kid. If you're uncertain of what size your toilet is, please research to understand if your toilet is definite round or elongated for the purpose of more info.

Travel Toilet Seats

You should have a backup strategy for your child while traveling. These types of travel toilet seats are excellent! They enable you to continue effective potty training for your son or daughter by assisting them to feel comfortable actually in a general public restroom. These types of travel toilet seats flip down could be put inside diaper handbags, purses or baggage. They can also be called Foldable Toilet Seats, and are available in multiple colors, designs, and personas. They are;

- ✓ Convenient to carry
- ✓ Easy to completely clean
- ✓ Light Weight
- ✓ Plenty of options in color, styles and character types

Be sure you provide extra clothing, underwear, and wipes upon brief or lengthy journeys in case your son or daughter has incidents.

Soft Toilet Seats:

Some children require extra cushioning while getting toilet training and even once they have perfected toilet schooling too. Ensuring your son or daughter is usually comfortable and seems secure makes all the difference through the toilet training procedure, and that is why gentle toilet seats are extremely important.

Whether you decide to make use of a toilet seat or a toilet chair, in any event, the kid must feel safe and sound with all the toilet. They need to have the ability to sit on the toilet easily in order to proceed to the toilet without feeling unpredictable within the toilet, or feeling like they could fall in; and using a toilet chair on the toilet can make all of the difference.

It has been discovered that children who have been toilet trained no longer want a toilet chair, but nonetheless, they do not fit correctly on the best toilet sometimes. The toilet seats should be the ideal size intended for children so they can fit easily on it.

Portable Potty Seats:

We provide a selection of lightweight toilet seats to choose from, so you as well as your kid can select the one which will continue to work best for all of them. We've picked the Toilet Patty or maybe the blue Toilet Scotty lightweight toilet seats that goes with the toilet teaching dolls. They are able to have the child's name put into the front side of them plus they are extremely long lasting and durable to make use of. They can fit comfortably together with the toilet and are extremely light-weight and easy to consider anywhere your son or daughter must move. There are also two other Toilet Patty and Toilet Scotty seats which have an easier style and can have your son or daughter's name put into all of them as well.

Along with these, gleam portable toilet chair is also foldable and incredibly much just like a real toilet for the reason that it fits very neatly around the toilet and there's a stage stool attached as well. This portable toilet seat will come in white and there are grips privately from the steps that can be mounted on to help kids experience secure hold on/off the toilet seat. There are several portable toilet seats you can expect, there are a lot more and you'll desire to look over them all to get the one that will continue to work right for you as well as your child

Chapter 7

How to Know if Toilet seat is certainly Circular or Elongated?

The most frequent residential toilet use to end up being round, particularly when space is tight, however, the trend is currently to elongated bowls.

Many commercial containers are elongated. Circular containers take up less space and are simpler to clean, and males have a tendency to choose elongated containers due to this extra space in front. An elongated dish is usually approximately two inches longer when compared to a round bowl. This leads to a bigger focus on the region and much less drip in the dish, as a result of enhancing hygienic conditions.

Dimensions are important if you are buying a new toilet seat.

Toilet Measurement to Determine Dish

✓ elongated (approximately 18.5" long).

✓ circular (approximately 16.5" long).

Measure from middle front side of dish to middle of the joint post openings (Not the Container). In the U. H., the typical range between joint post openings is 5.5". Go through the size of the fixture over.

Chapter 8

Methods for Effective Toilet Training

- Search for indicators of toilet schooling readiness prior to your jump in. Prior to you begin, you need to wait around until your baby displays indications of readiness. This typically consists of fewer damp diapers, desire for others using the toilet, verbalizing the actual fact that they are going to pee or feces, searching for a personal place to complete the job, and requesting to become transformed.

- Let your baby choose their particular own house training chair or seat. Permitting your child to truly have a say in the choice procedure can help infuse a feeling of empowerment and possession. We all recommend narrowing the options right down to a small number of appropriate options just before showing these to your child.

- Business lead by example. Kids are given birth to mimics, and viewing mom or father make use of the toilet depicts to them a moving picture that details all the potty-going procedure.

- Keep the scolding and put on the compliment. Accidents happen, again and again and once more. Because frustrating and reprimanding your baby might cause stress and lead improvement to a standstill. Instead of scolding your tot, claim that they get one of these little harder to get to the toilet the next time and make sure to be luxurious with compliment when the work gets carried out right. Kids crave authorization and are wanting to please, therefore be certain to prize employment done well with memorable actions like high fives, hugs, or perhaps a small triumph dance.

- Take a rest if necessary. Toilet training may be considered a roller-coaster trip of emotions, anticipations, and limitless cleanups. If you have tried almost everything and your kid still won't use a toilet or a toilet teaching chair, try going for a two-week break. Having a problem with your child is only going to make you both miserable and may even attract the procedure out much longer than necessary. Have a deep breathe and try once again when the waters are quiet.

Chapter 9

Types of Travel Potty

Certainly, one of the most crucial decisions you may make if you are looking to discover the best travel toilet is which kind you will use, as both types have got different benefits and drawbacks.

Stand-alone

A stand-alone travel toilet is precisely what it appears like, a toilet that stands alone. This sort of travel toilet is ideal for very long car journeys, as it enables your baby to visit the toilet wherever, whether in a remote wooded region or even in the rear of the car.

They include a very easily cleaned detachable container or a location for any bag to get your baby to visit in. As the clean-up is probably not everything much fun, this kind of travel potty is actually convenient.

Seat Just

Again, as the name implies, these types of travel potties are designed to fit over a normal toilet to permit your baby to take a seat on it with no falling in!

These seats aren't quite as easy, given that they have to be used in combination with a toilet, however they usually fold-up, making all of them a piece of cake to pack.

What to Remember When Investing in a Travel Toilet or Potty

Once you are buying any new kind of kid equipment, there are several things that you'll require to bear in mind. This is also true if you are searching to discover the best travel toilet.

Child's Choice

With regards to the age group of your son or daughter, you may want to look within a particular kind of chair. More youthful kids generally like the stand-alone kind of chair; this is for a few reasons, however, personally speaking, some are afraid of automated flushing lavatories, they wouldn't get close to them, significantly least take a seat on all of them while a few like it.

Be sure you take your child's opinion into consideration before you get or they will probably not want to use at all.

Secure

If you opt to get a chair only travel toilet, make sure to stay away from any that doesn't match the standard toilet chair. If it does not fit safely, there's a great chance that the chair will certainly slide and slip and dump your little poo off.

Obviously, this may be incredibly dangerous and may have a potentially harmful influence on your little toilet schooling experience.

Storage Space

A number of the stand-alone potties include space for storage on the edges, which may be utilized for wipes, paper, luggage, or tissues.

This is often true to lifesaver when you find out you loaded all that stuff in the bottom of the suitcase, which usually reaching underneath the stack might take time especially when your child needs to proceed at the moment!

Size

A number of toilet seats that are marketed to be used during travel are HUUUGE! Which usually, sort of causes them to be a little challenging to match right into a loaded car. Ensure that you look for a chair or seat that is the appropriate size for your baby.

Easy to Completely Clean

A term to the smart, be sure you have a small amount of water to use in case your child says they need to poo. It'll make an environment of difference if you are cleaning up their travel toilet!

Additionally, you want to make sure the fact that the toilet you decide on is simple to get rid of waste and to clean, or you'll spend a significant amount of period doing something gross rather than enjoying your holiday.

Foldable

In reducing the quantity of space adopted in either the trunk of your automobile or your suitcase, it could not be considered a bad idea to discover a travel potty chair that may be collapsed up. This can make this very much simpler to fit whenever you possess a supplementary little room.

Chapter 10

Ideas to Purchase a Toilet/Potty Training Seat for Your Kid

First of all, it is rather crucial to learn the difference between a potty-training chair and a potty seat. Second of all, choose equipment your son or daughter require and wish, and consider what exactly your requirements are concerning its use, cost, sturdiness, etc.

Even though a toilet chair is usually a stand-alone toilet gear, a toilet seat can be an attachable plastic material chair that fits on the standard mature toilet chair. Some children dread the adult toilet, which, subsequently, may hinder their learning process. That's the reason, many parents spend money on a toilet chair that is clearly a piece of low and comfy equipment meant for the infant.

Nevertheless, there are toddler-sized toilet seats, which can help the child sit easily on the mature toilet. One step potty could be of great help to climb and gain access to the chair and rest your toes on the step easily, instead of keeping all of them dangling.

The gear employed for the toilet training of the baby should not only end up being safe and comfortable designed for him, it should also be easy so that you can utilize it for a child. When this happens, a stand-alone chair can be considered a problem when compared with a toilet seat; you might have to do it again, the toilet chair cleaning process many times a day after every visit by a young child. Also, if you encounter issues which include difficulty in completely cleaning-up mess, the duty may become even more tedious and annoying.

On the other hand, if you select a youngsters' toilet seat, it will make them be associated with toilet teaching easily and practically because after the baby gets finished with his business, you merely have to remove it aside and you're done.

The potty chair must have a dial or a rubbery underside to avoid a child from slipping from the seat. This allows your child to match within the mature toilet flawlessly and decreases the chance of falling. In addition, it removes worries from the kid's brain of utilizing a larger toilet chair.

Usage of a splash safeguard will improve the toilet schooling by stopping the feasible clutter developed by a child if he/she is unable to go properly. Therefore, look at a toilet training chair with a dash safeguard, in the event that the kid seems unpleasant with all the splash safeguard, avoid this. Show patience enough to completely clean the clutter, and permit the kid to consider his time for you to learn to toilet train with no splash safeguard.

A toilet chair with deals over the edges is usually a much better option for small children, it can help the hold to seize the chair correctly when in a rush.

Some children may feel frightened of the whole toilet training point and could have a very long time to understand it. In order to avoid this, you make it possible for your child to select a toilet chair of his choice and wish that working out goes quicker along with his preferred equipment.

Whilst utilizing a kid-sized chair more than a grown-up toilet for your kid's house training, it's important to employ some step feces for just two factors: first of all, it could be frighteningly intended for your child to take a seat on an increased toilet chair, and second of all, when there are simply no step feces to press against, it could hamper his bowel motions.

Chapter 11

Benefits of Utilizing a Baby Potty Seat

Toilet teaching seat is one of the biggest innovations for simpler parenting and help prevent disastrous toilet training occurrences, and here are why skilled moms help you to purchase your toilet for your child -

✓ Waste materials could be easily cleaned/flushed hence decreases hassle.

✓ The transition to the adult toilet becomes organic and unforced and the children can quickly adjust to that.

✓ Credited to its light-weight feature, it is highly lightweighted and you may easily travel with it.

✓ Makes it simpler for children to make use of independently; decreases the necessity of these counting on you to visit.

- ✓ Its small size will not take up too much space round the house/toilet.

- ✓ It is children size and therefore helps it much less intimidating.

- ✓ Interactive features instantly attract children thus permits an easy toilet schooling experience

With so much benefits derived from the very best baby toilet chair; it is without a doubt a smart investment.

However, so many items on the market could be overwhelming to comprehend. Which greatest suits your need? did you get the best made potty training chair, the best travel potty or maybe the best convertible potty training chair?

Thus, simply by familiarizing, your using what each trainer provides will show you towards the merchandise that fulfills your needs. In the next section, we've reviewed ten of the greatest baby Potty Toilet Seats with their unique features and benefits and drawbacks to further help you with your questions.